Health Related Quality of

Pratima Sarwadikar
Shyam Ganvir

Health Related Quality of Life in elderly diabetic individuals

Association of physical activity, balance, gait speed on health related quality of life in elderly diabetic individuals

LAP LAMBERT Academic Publishing

Cover image: www.ingimage.com

Publisher:
LAP LAMBERT Academic Publishing
is a trademark of
International Book Market Service Ltd., member of OmniScriptum Publishing Group
17 Meldrum Street, Beau Bassin 71504, Mauritius

Printed at: see last page
ISBN: 978-620-0-50587-3

HEALTH RELATED QUALITY OF LIFE IN ELDERLY DIABETIC

INDIVIDUALS

1. Introduction

Ageing is associated with generalized slowing of movement. The ability to walk underlies many basic and community functions necessary for independence[12]. Walking requires multiple systems and organs support, such as central nervous system, peripheral nerves, bones and joints, muscles, heart and lungs, and blood. The capacity of walking can reflect the functions of organ systems.

Skeletal muscle mass and function decline with age, and this age-related deterioration of skeletal muscle is known as sarcopenia. The great challenge of aging is to maintain one's functional capacity, an individual's ability to independently carry out activities deemed essential. The decline in physical performance is inevitable, and gait speed is considered a global indicator of functional mobility. Reduced speed occurs with age even among the healthy elderly, and it has a significant impact on one's health and quality of life.

The change in gait speed is associated with physiological factors, behavioural factors, and the presence of diseases. It may also increase the risk of falling and result in disability, hospitalization, and death. Reduced speed is associated with the risk of poor health-related outcomes.

Mobility limitation, typically defined as difficulty walking one-quarter mile or climbing one flight of stairs, is reported by 30%–40% of older adults. Mobility limitation is a precursor to more severe mobility disability and increased dependence in daily activities, entry into nursing homes, and mortality. An emerging body of evidence supports the hypothesis that high energy requirements for daily activities, such as walking, play a central role in the development of mobility limitation among older adults. The energy cost of walking measures how much physiological work the body must perform during walking. Most healthy individuals have a preferred walking speed that minimizes their energy cost of walking. The energy cost of walking rises progressively with aging and is especially -high among older adults who report walking difficulty. a high energy cost of walking can have profound negative impacts on an older adult's overall mobility, causing decreases in the speed and quantity of movement. Reductions in the energy cost of walking could thus decrease fatigability and thereby increase daily physical activity, endurance, physical function, and life-space.

Geriatric is a medical term that encompasses the health of elderly patients. The definition of elderly, a perdon is considered as old if her civil age is ≥ 60 or 65 years old. While no specific age has been set for defining older adults, the general consensus considers the age of 60 years as a cut off (WHO 2015). Worldwide, the number of older adults aged 60 years and above is projected to increase from 841 million people in 2013 to more than 2 billion in 2050 (UN 2013). Most people over than 60 years old suffer from type 2 DM due to insulin resistance. However, insulin secretion may be severely reduced at the end stage of type 2 DM. Decreased physical performance, an important predictor of disability and functional decline, has been shown to have negative consequences on the daily life of older people. Diabetes is one of the major causes of physical limitation and individuals with diabetes have approximately 50–80% greater risk of disability compared to those without diabetes.

Successful aging encompasses multiple dimensions of health, including physical, functional, social, and psychological well-being. Maintaining a high level of quality of life into advanced age is a growing public health concern as the older adult population continues to increase. India has one of the highest prevalence of diabetes mellitus in the world (n ≥ 62 million). It is predicted that by 2030, 79.4 million individuals residing in India will suffer from the condition.

The prevention and good management of diabetes to reduce complications is thus of paramount importance. Indeed, several studies have under-lined the central role of physical activity in the management of type 1 or type 2 diabetes. In those with diabetes physical activity has been shown to improve glycaemic control, insulin sensitivity, and restore diabetes associated complications (cardiovascular disease and retinopathy). As ageing takes the physical ability goes lower, the elderly individuals feel worthless and obviously experience a significant obstacle before them in gaining life satisfaction from life. The reduced physiological capacity evident with ageing may affect the ability to perform many tasks, potentially affecting QoL. The physiological process of aging is marked by a decrease in motor skills, reduced strength, flexibility, speed and hindering daily activities and maintenance of a healthy lifestyle and ultimately decrease in QoL.

The primary types of diabetes are type 1 and type 2. Type 1 diabetes (5%–10% of cases) results from cellular-mediated autoimmune destruction of the pancreatic b-cells, producing insulin deficiency. Type 2 diabetes (90%–95% of cases) results from a progressive loss of insulin secretion, usually also with insulin resistance.

Type 2 diabetes is a major cause of morbidity and mortality and has become an important public health issue worldwide. Obesity and physical inactivity are well-known risk factors for the development of type 2 diabetes. Advances in socio-economic development, daily routines, changes in dietary habits, aging and sedentary life style have manifested into significant rise in number of patients suffering from diabetes mellitus, Diabetes has become global health problem and its complications have led to rise in mortality and morbidity. As the number of patients suffering from diabetes is increasing, it has become very essential to quantify the prevalence so that resources are allocated properly.

NEED FOR THE STUDY:

Aging or aging is the process of becoming older. In humans, ageing represents the accumulation of changes in a human being over time including physical, psychological, and social changes. Ageing is among the greatest known risk factors for the most human diseases. Healthy ageing has been defined as an ability to lead a healthy, socially inclusive lifestyle relatively free from illness or disability, and this is more likely in those actively engaging in activities to improve their health and wellbeing.

The results of this study suggest that balance impairments are present in people with diminished confidence in their balance ability and play an important role in determining balance confidence. This relationship has important implications for the development of rehabilitation programs that aim to improve balance confidence and diminish its impact on function in elderly people. An in-depth understanding of the predictors of balance confidence is necessary to identify and effectively manage those people at risk for declining balance confidence, and possibly prevent the decline of function that is a consequence of this pervasive problem in elderly people.

The measurement of gait speed is considered a simple and effective measure for evaluating the functional capacity of elderly people. There is growing interest in applying the gait velocity (GV) measurement as a simple test in ambulatory clinics to detect mobility problems and to predict adverse outcomes in the elderly population.

Although previous studies have shown that gait disorders and impairment in GV could predict adverse events in disabled elderly persons, it is still uncertain whether this single measurement

5

of physical performance is enough to predict health outcomes in high functioning older persons.

Populations with low incomes, ethnic minorities and older people with disabilities are the most likely to be inactive. Policies and programmes should encourage inactive people to become more active as they age and to provide them with opportunities to do so. It is particularly important to provide safe areas for walking and to support culturally-appropriate community activities that stimulate physical activity and are organized and led by older people themselves. Professional advice to "go from doing nothing to doing something" and physical rehabilitation programmes that help older people recover from mobility problems are both effective and cost-efficient. (WHO, 1998). The great challenge of aging is to maintain one's functional capacity, an individual's ability to carry out physical activities independently.

The of study is planned to gather information of physical activity and balance to clarify the relationship between physical activity and balance om maximal gait speed in community dwelling older adults.

The purpose of this study, First, we would like to address the nature of the Physical activity and balance in community dwelling older adults. Second, to find out the relationship of physical activity and balance on maximal gait speed.

Types of diabetes mellitus and the mechanism

Type 1 diabetes

In type 1 diabetes there is autoimmune destruction of the pancreas leading to a failure to secrete insulin. Although trials are underway to explore the prevention of this process, it is at present a relentless and chronic disorder. It represents the most common endocrinological disease of childhood affecting as many as 1 in 500 children under 18, and the incidence would appear to be increasing.1 Exogenous insulin is essential in the treatment of this condition and represents the only available treatment for approximating normal physiology.

Since the introduction of insulin in the 1920s, when treatment was aimed at preventing ketoacidosis, the process of insulin administration has become more elaborate with increasing varieties and techniques. The aims of treatment for a diabetic now include mimicry of normal insulin levels throughout the day, achieving tight control, and prevention of microvascular and macrovascular complications.

RISKS OF EXERCISE IN TYPE 1 DIABETES

The major risks to the exercising type 1 diabetic subject are potentially life threatening metabolic disturbances and the associated morbidity and mortality of microvascular and macrovascular complications. Despite the best precautions, hypoglycaemia can occur, and, although moderate exercise itself may not mask hypoglycaemic responses in patients with type 1 diabetes, during vigorous activity this feedback may be impaired,11 with additional orthostatic hypotension, impaired thermoregulaton, and neuropathy confusing the hypoglycaemic symptoms.12 These may be worse in the morning,13 and all patients with type 1 diabetes should carry rapidly absorbable high glycaemic carbohydrates/drinks, glucagon, or "Hypostop". The normal alcohol consumption that occurs after a game in many sports can also pose additional risks of exercise induced hypoglycaemia with a failure to recognise the warnings, occasionally seen as a problem in subaqua divers where "nitrogen narcosis" and exercise induced hypoglycaemia produce interchangeable symptoms.

Post-exercise hypoglycaemia and delayed onset hypoglycaemia can occur up to four and 24 hours after exercise respectively. The increased insulin sensitivity and depleted glycogen stores conspire to produce profound hypoglycaemia, most commonly nocturnal.14 This neuroglycopenia has been suggested to disturb sleep patterns, alter recovery, and therefore affect physical performance the following day and carries significant morbidity and mortality. Recent studies in this department have shown that one hour of nocturnal hypoglycaemia reduces the sense of wellbeing and increases subjective determinants of fatigue but produces no alterations in the hormonal, glucose, and lactate response to exercise. Interestingly, cerebral, cardiovascular, and physical performance also show no objective alterations.15 For the person concerned, nocturnal hypoglycaemia nevertheless remains an alarming risk, and an evening snack or reduced evening dose of insulin after activity may be warranted. Hyperglycaemia as discussed above produces both acute and long term consequences, increasing the risks of cardiovascular disease, sudden death, reduced exercise capacity, hypertension, retinopathy, nephropathy, and neuropathy, which can all significantly worsen with impaired control.

Type 2 diabetes

Type 2 diabetes (formerly known as noninsulin dependent diabetes mellitus) occurs almost exclusively in the adult population and its main feature is insulin resistance, manifested as hyperinsulinaemia and hyperglycaemia. It is strongly correlated with obesity, physical inactivity, and family history and accounts for 90% of all diabetes. Typically as many as 80% are overweight and many are elderly.

PHYSIOLOGY OF EXERCISE AND TRAINING IN IMPAIRED GLUCOSE TOLERANCE AND TYPE 2 DIABETES

Many of the extreme changes in metabolism seen in type 1 diabetes are blunted. Instead hyperinsulinism and hyperglycaemia are present concurrently because of the preservation of pancreatic â-cell function and hepatic and skeletal muscle insulin resistance, with hypoglycaemia therefore relatively uncommon. The initial presentation of type 2 diabetes is as insulin resistance, an impaired response to endogenous insulin, and therefore impaired glucose tolerance. As with type 1 diabetes, exercise produces increased glucose uptake in skeletal muscle. Unlike in type 1 diabetes, however, those with type 2 diabetes are able to produce significant decreases in ambient blood glucose and insulin concentrations without increasing the risk of hypoglycaemia. This is due in part to reduced hepatic glucose production but mainly to increased muscle glucose uptake through increased delivery, oxidation, and storage of carbohydrates. In type 2 diabetes, this increased uptake appears to bypass the normal regulation at rest and promotes increased glucose uptake for up to several hours with a concomitant fall in glycaemia. A single exercise bout has been shown to increase insulin sensitivity in liver and muscle for up to hours while prolonged exercise produces a fall in hyperglycaemia and hyperinsulinaemia. Initially athletes were noticed to have reduced plasma glucose and insulin concentrations in response to oral glucose loading, with the suggestion that exercise improved insulin sensitivity. The increase in insulin sensitivity with exercise has since been well established, and controlled studies of exercise intervention/training have resulted in improved insulin sensitivity, increased carbohydrate oxidation, and reductions in body mass. Hughes *et al*, showed an improvement in insulin sensitivity with training at 50–70% VO2MAX, and many studies have reported immediate changes in total glucose disposal and skeletal muscle uptake. In subjects who trained vigorously, improvements in glucose disposal were double for up to 10 days. These beneficial effects of training unfortunately appear to be transient, declining after seven days and 10 days, and are in part derived from increased GLUT4 transporter recruitment, which has also been shown to be higher in athletes56 and after training. In addition, exercise and training promote increased blood flow, insulin receptor, and oxidative and non-oxidative enzyme concentrations in muscle. Although aerobic training also promotes the transition to a greater percentage of type 1 and 2a muscle fibres, the importance of this is not fully understood. Instead the preservation of the lean body tissues, in particular muscle mass, and the reductions in fat mass appear to be significant contributors to improved insulin sensitivity.

Criteria to check for the existence of type II DM in adults (adapted from the American Diabetes Association.

1. Subjects aged more than 45 years (When normal, the checkup should be repeated every 1–3 years)

2. Occurrence of symptoms like polyuria, polydipsia, and unexplained weight loss

3. Asymptomatic subjects carrying at least one of the following risk factors:

3.1. Have a first-degree parent with diabetes

3.2. Overweight or with a BMI >25 kg/m2

3.3. History of impaired glucose tolerance or impaired fasting glucose in a previous test

3.4. Hypertension (>140/90 mmHg)

3.5. A plasma high density lipoprotein cholesterol level <35 mg/ dl and/or a plasmatic triglyceride level >250 mg/dl

3.6. History of gestational DM or of a newborn child weighing more than 4.08 kg

3.7. Sedentary lifestyle

3.8. Other clinical conditions associated with insulin resistance, such as polycystic ovary syndrome and acanthosis nigricans.

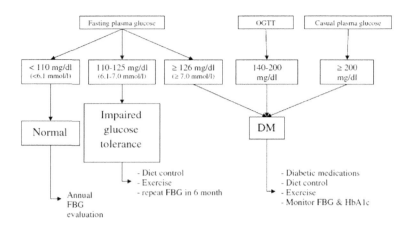

Figure: Guidelines for diagnosis of diabetic mellitus in individuals

Diabetes mellitus is a chronic metabolic disease characterized by hyperglycaemia and high glycated haemoglobin with or without glycosuria. Diabetes was diagnosed according to any one of the following criteria:

Table: Normal and Abnormal Values for OGTT and FPG

FPG Values	OGTT Values	Remarks
FPG < 100mg/dl (5.6 mmol/l)	2-h postload glucose < 140 mg/dl (7.8 mmol/l)	Normal glucose tolerance
FPG < 100-125 mg/dl(5-6-6.9 mmol/l)	2-h postload glucose 140-199 mg/dl (7.8-11.1 mmol/l)	Impaired glucose tolerance
FPG < 126 mg/dl (7.0 mmol/l)	2-h postload glucose > 200 mg/dl (11.1 mmol/l)	Provisional diaganosis of Diabetes

Impaired glucose intolerance is associated with aging, and postprandial hyperglycemia is a prominent characteristic of type 2 diabetes in older adults. Age-related insulin resistance is associated with changes in body composition and physical inactivity among other factors, which may partially explain the greatest relative benefits of the intensive lifestyle intervention observed among older participants.

Diabetes mellitus mechanism

Normal blood glucose control

AT REST

Blood glucose concentrations must be maintained within narrow limits. This is essential to prevent the acute and chronic complications seen in diabetes mellitus4 and is achieved through a balance between the processes that add and remove glucose from the normal circulation. In the fasting state, glucose is produced by the liver and closely balances the uptake and losses into body tissues, responding closely to the circulating plasma glucose concentrations. In the postprandial state glucose is absorbed through the alimentary system, causing a rise in blood glucose concentrations. Insulin is released which reduces hepatic glucose production and increases the disposal of glucose in peripheral tissue, thus reducing blood glucose. Some 90% of this clearance occurs through increased uptake in skeletal muscle where glucose is transported into muscle by facilitated diffusion. This occurs through the translocation of a family of transporter proteins to the membrane surface, almost all of which are the GLUT4 transporter. A limited number of GLUT5 transporters are also present which allow relatively slow fructose transport.

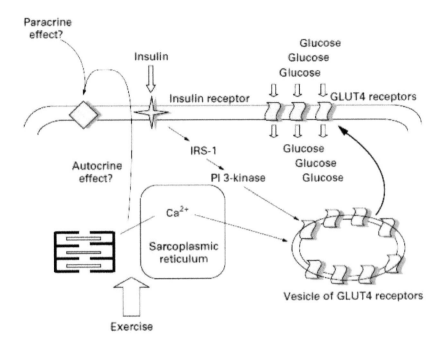

DURING EXERCISE

During exercise the large changes in energy utilisation require fine adjustments of glucose and non-esterified fatty acid concentrations within the blood. During the first 5–10 minutes of moderate intensity exercise, glycogen provides the major fuel source for skeletal muscle, but as exercise duration is prolonged, the contribution of plasma (blood borne) glucose and non-esterified fatty acid predominates. To match this increased demand, a complex hormonal and autonomic response allows an increase in hepatic glucose production and tissue uptake while increasing mobilisation of non-esterified fatty acid from adipose tissue deposits. This is produced both by a fall in circulating insulin concentrations and a wide variety of "counter-regulatory" hormones, increased secretion of which counters the hypoglycaemic action of insulin. Elevations in the blood concentrations of these hormones, which include adrenaline, glucagon, cortisol, and growth hormone, promote both increased glucose production and mobilisation of nonesterified fatty acids from adipose storage sites. In addition, production of new glucose in the liver (gluconeogenesis) from substrates such as lactate is enhanced. Direct sympathetic stimulation of the pancreas and liver after muscle contraction may also bypass initial hormonal control, and additional fuel supplies are provided by ketone formation and mobilisation of lactate from inactive muscle glycogen. Glucose transport into muscle is again provided by the transporter protein GLUT4, but the protein is recruited to the membrane surface in large quantities in contracting muscle, independently of insulin (fig 1). Together these changes maintain the increased fuel supply for exercising muscle and prevent hypoglycaemia from excessive utilisation.

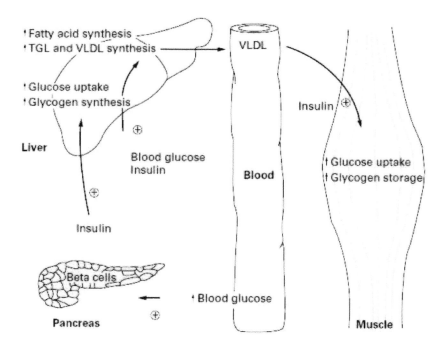

AFTER EXERCISE

At the end of exercise the body in essence enters a fasted state in which glycogen stores in muscle and liver are low and hepatic glucose production is accelerated. The counterregulatory hormone levels may remain elevated for some considerable time and there is a concomitant hyperglycaemic and hyperinsulinaemic response. Glycogen resynthesis in the muscle occurs at first largely as a result of increased GLUT4 transport and insulin sensitivity and without the need for insulin. At a variable time point later, as homoeostasis is reached and glycogen, glucose, and hormone levels return to normal, insulin may be required to produce additional glucose uptake and glycogen resynthesis in muscle and liver. In the insulin deficient or resistant state, storage of glucose may therefore be impaired within muscle because of incomplete transport and decreased glycogen synthase activity.

Elderly type 2 DM is apparently due to several mechanisms among which one can cite genetic background, long life expectancy leading to decrease in insulin secretion, and the modification of some environmental factors responsible for the comorbidities in elderly. The lack of physical activity added to eating disorders characterizing modern life style is the most incriminated factors.

Symptoms and positive diagnosis of diabetes mellitus in elderly

Common symptoms leading to DM diagnosis are complications such as neuropathy or nephropathy, heart, heart and vascular problems and/or recurrent urinary infections or skin problems.

Fatigue, hypotension, incontinence, cognitive impairment of functional decline, depression, and dementia that might be the first manifestations of the disease are usually wrongly attributed to aging.

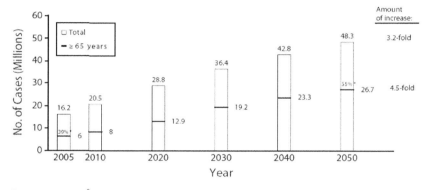

Source. Narayan et al.[6]

FIGURE 1—Projected number of cases of diagnosed diabetes among total population and older adults aged 65 years and older: United States, 2005-2050.

Exercise prescription in Type 2 diabetes

Current guidelines from the American Diabetes Association (ADA), the European Association for the Study of Diabetes (EASD) or the American College of Physicians (ACP) all acknowledge the therapeutic strength of exercise intervention. The ADA states that 'to improve glycemic control, assist with weight maintenance, and reduce risk of CVD, at least 150 min/week of moderate- intensity aerobic physical activity is recommended and/ or at least 90 min/week of vigorous aerobic exercise, distributed over at least 3 days/week and with no more than 2 consecutive days without physical activity.' Since 2006, the ADA guidelines explicitly mention and recognize that 'in the absence of contraindications, people with Type 2 diabetes should be encouraged to perform resistance exercise 3 times a week, targeting all major muscle groups, progressing to 3 sets of 8–10 repetitions at a weight that can not be lifted more than 8–10 times. Diet and exercise therapy form the basis of treatment of type 2 diabetes mellitus (T2DM). These two approaches are well known to improve blood glucose control. Exercise therapy has also been reported to be effective in improving blood glucose control and quality of life (QOL). However, reduction of fat and improvement in insulin resistance are limited with diet modification alone.

"Perform moderate-intensity exercise (approximately 3 METs)"

    (i) Perform moderate-intensity exercise for at least 20 minutes per day.
    (ii) Set the target for the number of steps at 8000 steps or more.
    (iii) Do not exercise too strenuously on a day on which you do not feel
        well.

← Specific targets for exercise

"What kind of exercise is moderate-intensity exercise (approximately 3 METs)?"

Recommended exercise is quick walking. The walking speed at which while talking you feel a little strenuous is appropriate.

Quick walking (speed: approximately 70 to 90 m/min)

Note: the average walking speed of elderly people (65 years of age or older) is "approximately 55 m/min."

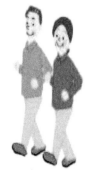

Walking

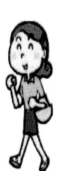

Shopping

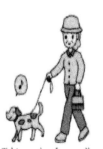

Taking a dog for a walk

← Examples of 3 METs

Public Policy

Appropriate public policies can increase the availability and accessibility of services for older adults with diabetes.

The following 5 public policy efforts can help improve health care services for older diabetic Americans:

1. Facilitate coordination of services to older diabetic patients to eliminate service redundancy and increase patients' use of existing services. The coordination of services is particularly important for noninstitutionalized patients, especially women, who often live alone and in poverty.

2. Expand the delivery of in-home health care by using combinations of health professionals and lay people to provide services.

3. Expand diabetes education to include people serving as caregivers for older adults with diabetes, including training on how to interface with health professionals in providing care.

4. Ensure that standard medical care provided to older adults with diabetes includes formal systematic assessments of their physical, emotional, and social functioning so that any barriers to appropriate self-care can be identified and, if possible, overcome.

5. Promote analytic modeling of the efficacy and cost-effectiveness of interventions specifically designed to help older Americans with diabetes. An area to consider is assessing the interventions to address geriatric syndromes by estimating constructs such as disability-free life expectancy, an approach similar to the concepts of compression of morbidity and active aging.

Physical Activity

An important determinant of quality of life is physical activity. Apart from lowering physical fitness and performance, insufficient physical activity can also increase the risk of muscle atrophy, sarcopenia, osteoporosis, type 2 diabetes, arterial hypertension, coronary heart disease, and certain types of cancer in elder individuals. Physical activity includes all movement that increases energy use, whereas exercise is planned, structured physical activity. Physical activity: Bodily movement produced by the contraction of skeletal muscle that requires energy expenditure in excess of resting energy expenditure. A physically active lifestyle is important for the prevention and treatment of many chronic diseases and conditions. Exercise improves blood glucose control in type 2 diabetes, reduces cardiovascular risk factors, contributes to weight loss, and improves well-being. Higher physical activity (PA) has been associated with concrete health benefits, such as reduced risk for certain types of cancer, obesity, metabolic syndrome, T2D, CVD, and all-cause mortality. Increased PA is associated both with improved physical performance and change in body composition. Higher levels of PA appear to be associated with better functioning and better HRQoL.

Physical activity (PA) can play a major role in preventing multi morbidity in this age group because of the wide range of health conditions which can be positively influenced by PA. Regular PA in older adults contributes to a variety of health benefits such as lower risks of cardiovascular diseases, functional limitations, dementia and all-cause mortality as well as better psychological wellbeing. PA plays an important role in the treatment and management of many chronic diseases and conditions such as hypertension, hyperlipidaemia, type 2 diabetes and obesity. Daily physical activity. We measured daily self-reported occupational, household, and leisure physical activities over the past 7 days using the Physical Activity Scale for the Elderly from 0 to 400.

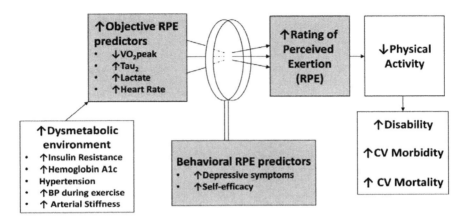

Fihure2: Conceptual model of perceived effort during exercise.

Physical inactivity is that it leads to reductions in lean muscle mass and strength. The reduction of muscle mass and strength to levels below proposed thresholds results in limitations in physical functioning and mobility, and reduces the opportunity for independent living in later life. Participation in physical activity (PA) promotes healthy aging and plays an important role in improving quality of life (QoL) among elderly.

Fear of fall

Falling is a common problem associated with aging. Although serious injuries such as hip fractures and wrist fractures are a well-recognized consequence of falls, the fear of falling is thought to be a more pervasive problem in the elderly population. When compared with other common fears, fear of falling ranked first among elderly people living in the community. Developing a fear of falling is more prevalent with increasing age and fall history. The impact of fear of falling is far-reaching because it can lead to activity restriction and diminished mobility, with as many as 56% of elderly people curtailing activities due to this fear.

What is quality of life?

It is a standard level that consists of the expectations of an individual or society for a good life. It is a subjective, multidimensional concept that defines a standard level of emotional, physical and social wellbeing. QOL is a broad ranging concept and there is no universally accepted definition of QOL is perceived as a state of well-being. World Health Organization (WHO) defines QOL as individuals perception of their position in life in the context of the culture and value systems in which they live in relation to their goals, expectations, standards and concerns". When quality of life is considered in the context of health and disease, it is commonly referred to as health-related quality of life (HRQoL) to differentiate it from other aspects of quality of life.

Defining QoL has proven challenging and many approaches to defining quality of life exist. There are approaches based on human needs, subjective well-being, expectations, and phenomenological viewpoints. A related literature on well-being distinguishes between approaches based on objective lists, preference satisfaction, hedonism, flourishing, and life satisfaction. Examples of definitions of QoL are: "a conscious cognitive judgment of satisfaction with one's life" and "an individuals' perception of their position in life in the context of the culture and value systems in which they live and in relation to their goals, expectations, standards and concerns"

Quality of Life Research Objectives

• To assess overall treatment efficacy, including subjective morbidity

• To help determine whether the goals of treatment have been met

• To educate patients and clinicians about the full spectrum of treatment outcomes

• To facilitate medical decision making

• To provide the defining issue if treatments are otherwise equivalent

• To compare outcomes across treatments and populations

What is Health related quality of life?

Health is fundamental to human life. The World Health Organization (WHO), in its constitution, has defined health as "A state of complete physical, mental, and social well-being not merely the absence of disease or infirmity". Leading health organizations has also identified HRQOL as a goal for people across all life stages. Use of HRQOL instruments have been incorporated in health surveillance and are considered valid indicators for health needs, policy documents, service requirements and intervention outcomes. Development and utilization of HRQOL instruments increased in last decade in efforts to improve patient health and value of health care services. Participation in physical activity (PA) promotes healthy aging and plays an important role in improving quality of life (QoL) among elderly.

The use of HRQOL studies is suitable in understanding effect of interventions on different populations. Physical, social and emotional impact of diseases and their impact on patients' lives are focus of HRQOL studies. Quality of life is frequently measured in investigations to evaluate the health of both clinical and general populations, and is therefore termed health related quality of life (HRQL). QoL is related to an individual's perception of the position in life in the context of culture and value systems and is influenced in a complex way by the person's physical health, psychological state, level of independence, and social relationships. Health-related quality of life (HRQoL) is part of a multidimensional approach that considers physical, mental, and social aspects

The quantification of HRQOL broadly separated into generic and disease-specific. The primary application of HRQOL measures is clinical evaluation but it has also been applied to health planning, population monitoring, health service research and policy evaluation. One potential limitation of biomedical measures is that it may not, sometimes, indicate improvement in health function and status. Incorporation of HRQOL measure to assess physical, psychological and social functioning complements the outcome and assessment derived from biomedical measures. Vitality, pain and cognitive function are also important domains of HRQOL. Generic instruments are applied to measure HRQOL across various health conditions. Disease specific instruments are used to measure a specific disease or group of diseases.

There are, however, few studies that have examined the association between physical activity and health related quality of life in elderly among the rural population. Since these are important factors that promote optimal health in elderly, studying the association between PA and HRQoL is becoming more essential, especially as the number of elderly is increasing. This study assesses the association between PA and HRQoL in community dwelling elderly (≥ 60 years old). The purpose of this study to find out the association between the physical activity and health related quality of life in elderly among rural population.

Walking Speed

Walking is a measure of physical function which is related to musculoskeletal strength and power and is vital for independent life at higher ages. GV was measured as the time taken to walk the middle 8 meters of 10 meters and was timed by a chronometer. The first and last meters, considered as warm-up and deceleration phases, respectively, were not included in the calculation. Participants began the GV test on the word ''go'' and were instructed to ''walk at a comfortable and secure pace.'' Each participant performed the task twice after one non timed practice trial. The final score was the time in seconds of the quicker of two timed trials.

SEDENTARY LIFESTYLE

Sedentary behavior refers to the tendency to sit during waking hours with low energy expenditures. The mean sitting time is estimated to be approximately 6-7 h/d in developed countries, and a decreased level of physical activity has been shown to be inversely associated with increased sitting time.

DAILY PHYSICAL ACTIVITY

Daily physical activity is defined as continuous bodily movements via the contraction of skeletal muscle that results in an increase in energy expenditure in daily life. This includes various activities that are conducted in both occupational and leisure time such as walking, working at a desk, washing, cooking, and sports. On the other hand, exercise is defined as planned, structured, and repetitive physical activity that has the objective of improving physical fitness. Physical activity is usually classified by its intensity and duration. The metabolic equivalent (MET) is a useful measurement for representing the intensity of physical activity and is defined as the amount of oxygen uptake while sitting at rest. An oxygen uptake of 3.5 mL/kg per minute is equal to the basal resting metabolic rate and is considered to be 1 MET.

WALKING

Walking is one of the most common physical activities of daily life. However, 54.6% of patients with T2D have reported engaging in no weekly physical activity through walking], demonstrating that patients with T2D should walk more frequently.

NON-EXERCISE ACTIVITY THERMOGENESIS

Daily physical activity, with the exception of volitional sports-like activities, is defined as non-exercise activity thermogenesis (NEAT). NEAT is the main determinant of variability in total daily energy expenditure, which varies substantially from person to person by up to 2000 kcal/d. NEAT is influenced by various factors. For example, NEAT has been shown to increase by 25% seven days after a single bout of high-intensity walking exercise. Moreover, regular exercise, especially moderate- to vigorous-intensity exercise, may increase NEAT; in contrast, living in an urban area populated with individuals who live a sedentary lifestyle will likely result in a decrease in NEAT.

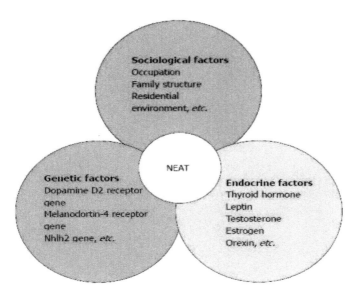

Figure 1 **Non-exercise activity thermogenesis is intricately regulated by sociological, endocrinological, and genetic factors.** NEAT: Non-exercise activity thermogenesis.

Aim

The aim of this study to find out the association of physical activity and health related quality of life in elderly diabetic individuals from rural community

Objectives

- To assess the physical activity in elderly diabetic individuals.
- To assess the health related quality of life in elderly diabetic individuals.

Materials and Methodology

- **Sample size:** 10 (Both male and female)
- **Study design:** A cross-sectional Study
- **Study duration:** 3 months
- **Sampling method:** Convenient sampling
- **Target Population:** Elderly with diabetic
- **Study setting:** Primary Health Centre and Tertiary Health Centres
- **Ethical considerations:** The study proposal approved for the ethical clearance from the institutional ethics committee. Prior to data collection and assessment informed consent was obtained from each subjects.

Eligibility criteria

Inclusion criteria

a. Age of more than 60 years
b. Either sex
c. Diabetes patients
   (1) fasting plasma glucose $\geq$ 126 mg/dl (7.0 mmol/l),

(2) 2-hours plasma glucose ≥ 200 mg/dl (11.1 mmol/l) during an oral glucose tolerance test.

d. Absence of cognitive and perceptual problems

e. A history of at least 6 months residing in nursing home for old people who were in this group

Exclusion criteria

a. Previous history of angina, severe vascular disease, any neurological disorders.

b. Patients with neuropathy and/ or hypothyroidism, liver diseases.

c. Patients with a history of drug or alcohol abuse.

d. Patients with mental, communication, and behavioural disorders that may cause problems in understanding or answering the questions.

e. Any recent surgeries

Outcomes

1.Physical activity was assessed by physical activity scale for elderly.

The PASE scores consist of three types of physical activities. However, the psychometric properties of these scores derived from leisure, household and work-related physical activities. The PASE-C is a 12-item scale for estimating the older adults' lifestyle physical activities, including three types of physical activity, such as leisure-time activity (5 items: walking, light/moderate/strenuous sport and recreational activities, and muscle strength), household activity (6 items: light housework, heavy house chores, home repairs, lawn work/yard care, outdoor gardening, and caring for another person), and work-related activity (1 item: work for pay or as volunteer). Scores of leisure-time, household and work-related physical activities were computed respectively, which were estimated by multiplying the amount of time spent (never, seldom [1-2 days], sometimes [3-4 days], and often [5-7 days]) in each activity by item weights and summed based on the scoring manual instructions. Scores range from 0 to 400. The tool is designed to assess household, occupational and leisure activity items.

The Physical Activity Scale for the Elderly (PASE) is an easily administered and scored instrument that measures the level of physical activity in individuals aged 65 years and older. The PASE can be used to measure physical activity levels in epidemiologic surveys of older people as well as to assess the effectiveness of exercise interventions. The leisure activity items require respondents to first report the number of days per week the activity was performed and then the number of hours per day. The reliability of PASE scores was evaluated by stability over repeated administrations three to seven weeks apart. PASE scores are calculated from weights and frequency values for each of 12 types of activity. The test-retest reliability coefficient was .75 (95% CI = .69-.80).

2.Health Related Quality of life assessed with SF-36 Questionnaire.

Health-related QoL, The Medical Outcomes Survey Short Form-36 (MOS SF- 36) questionnaire was administered to assess HRQL over the previous four weeks. The MOS SF-36 is a widely used, reliable, and valid criterion measure of HRQL in numerous populations. The MOS SF-36 questionnaire has 36 questions that are scored to measure eight domains of HRQL pertaining to both physical and mental health. The domains of physical functioning, role limitations due to physical health (role-physical), bodily pain, and general health comprised the physical component of HRQL, whereas the domains of vitality, social functioning, role limitations due to emotional health (role-emotional), and mental health comprised the mental component of HRQL. Each domain was scored using a scale ranging between 0 and 100, with higher scores indicating a higher HRQL than lower scores. Internal consistency of the MOS SF-36 is good.

Operational Definitions:

- Quality of life: Quality of life as individual perceptions of life in the context of local culture and value systems, as well as in relation to goals, expectations, standards and concerns.

- Physical activity: Bodily movement produced by the contraction of skeletal muscle that requires energy expenditure in excess of resting energy expenditure.

- Health: WHO has defined health as a dynamic state of physical, psychological, social and spiritual well-being and not just an absence of infirmity.

- Healthy ageing has been defined as an ability to lead a healthy, socially inclusive lifestyle relatively free from illness or disability, and this is more likely in those actively engaging in activities to improve their health and wellbeing

- Health related quality of life: HRQL is defined as an individuals' perspective of well-being in physical, mental and social domains of life

- Diabetes mellitus: Diabetes mellitus is "a group of diseases marked by high levels of blood glucose resulting from defects in insulin production, insulin action, or both.

Data Analysis:

The demographic data was analysed by the mean, median and standard deviation. unpaired t test was used to test the significance in quantitative variables. The association between the physical activity and health related quality of life analysed and P value shows <0.0001 is considered significant.

Table 1: Mean and Standard Deviation of PASE Score and HRQoL Score

Score	Mean	SD
PASE score	86.35	29.24
HRQoL Score	540.09	56.45

*CI= 95%, P value <0.0001 significant

Procedure:

After obtaining the ethical approval from the ethical committee, started the recruiting the participants from the primary, secondary and tertiary health care centres and from the diabetic clinic located in the rural area. Participants selected according to the inclusion and exclusion criteria, after that baseline characteristics of the participants were assessed. Physical activity and the health related quality of life of the selected participants were assessed by the selected instruments. Data of the all the participants were collected, analysed and result was calculated.

Result:

Table 2 shows the Socio-demographic and the components of the physical and the domains of the quality of life of the respondents. The mean age of the respondents 68.1 years including all the respondents were diagnosed with diabetic mellitus. All the respondents showed lower values in strenuous sports and heavy household work in the Physical activity scale. On the health related quality of life all the respondents showed decreased score in the energy/fatigue and the health change domains.

Table 3 shows the association between the physical activity score and the Health related quality of life (SF-36 score). On the analysis, adequate physical activity is most strongly associated with age and those who do daily activities like household activities, grooming, leisure's activities independently and regularly. Health related quality of life in diabetic respondents were associated with the age and the daily physical activities. As the age increases it may affect physical activities and the quality of life of the respondents.

Graph 1 shows the association between physical activity and the health related quality of life related to age. This graph shows that as the age increases the daily activities of the respondents may decrease because of the lower muscular strength or the any associated diseases like Diabetes Mellitus, Hypertension etc. Physical activities of all the respondents also decreases because of the living in the rural area, the living independently, poverty etc. and the quality life of that such respondents also changes as the physical activity decreases.

This study indicated statistically significant association between the adequate physical activity and the domains of health related quality of life such as energy/fatigue and the health changes because of the inadequate or routine hospital check-up in the rural population.

Table 2: Socio-demograpghic data and The Domains of PASE Scale and SF-36 Questionnaire.

Characteristics	Mean values
N	10
Age	68.1
Gender	Male(66.5), Female(70.5)
• **PASE Activity**	**Score**
Walking (h/day)	15.5
Light sports (h/day)	6.69
Moderate sports (h/day)	6.7
Strenuous sports (h/day)	**5.29**
Muscular strength/endurance (h/day)	11.85
Outdoor gardening (%)	11
Light housework (%)	10.5
Heavy housework (%)	**6.15**
Home repair (%)	8.25
Lawn work/yard care (%)	12.42
• **HRQoL (SF-36) Domains**	**Score**
Physical functioning	79.5
Role limitation due to physical health	59.5
Role limitation due to emotional problem	76.69

Energy/Fatigue	**51**
Emotional well-being	60.4
Social functioning	55
Pain	55
General health	55.5
Health change	**47.5**

Table 3: Association between PASE activity score and HRQoL(SF-36) score

Sr.No	Age/Gender	PASE Score	SF-36 Score
1	60	138	643.5
2	62	108	607.5
3	63	106.05	572.2
4	65	101.75	551.2
5	65	97.2	532.7
6	69	81.05	529.7
7	70	61.95	510.2
8	71	65.7	508.7
9	74	66.05	496.5
10	75	37.8	448.7

Graph 1: Association Between Physical Activity Scale and Health Related Quality Of Life with age

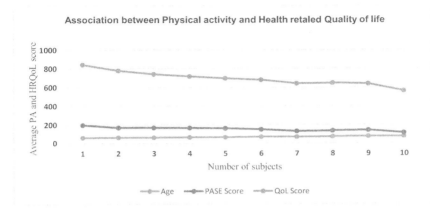

Association between Physical activity and Health retaled Quality of life

Discussion

The primary findings of this investigation were that healthy older adults who participated in regular physical activity of at least moderate intensity for more than one hour per week had higher values in all eight domains of HRQL than those who were less physically active.

This study aimed to evaluate the association between physical activity in elderly HRQoL who were independent older people living in a rural area. The elderly was included in this study as their HRQoL evaluated because their functional level could affect the quality of life. Most participants in the study, thought that regular physical activity was important to control diabetes. Physical activity in the control of diabetes was thought to be more important for men and women for those above the 65 years of age.

The finding of this study and the previous literatures shows findings in populations of people with diabetes residing in other locations, relating to the awareness of physical activity benefits. Brassill et al.[10] (2010) found in a sample of 115 people with diabetes residing in Ireland that 90% reported an awareness of the benefits of exercise in diabetes control. These data suggest that those with diabetes are indeed aware of the benefits of physical activity yet this awareness does not seem to translate into a high prevalence of physical activity.

Other studies have shown that organized, high-intensity exercise regimens can benefit HRQoL in both diseased and healthy populations.[11] This study extends these findings by showing that the less nature of physical activity is positively related to multiple domains of HRQL in healthy older adults. An active lifestyle preserves physical function in older adults, which may possibly contribute to higher levels of HRQoL scores in domains related to physical health.

Exercise therapy is essential for the management of diabetes. A sedentary lifestyle is known to be a major risk factor of cardiovascular disease (CVD). The American College of Sports Medicine and the American Diabetes Association have recommended at least 150 min/wk of moderate (50%-70% of an individual's maximum heart rate) to vigorous (> 70% of an individual's maximum heart rate) physical activity for patients with type 2 diabetes (T2D).

In a selected older adult, physical activity level was associated with less with energy/fatigue and health changes but not with the other domains of HRQoL. It is possible that the range in physical activity level was too narrow within the sedentary older adults, thereby limiting the influence that physical activity may have exerted on HRQL domains. The present study supports that, as the group having higher physical activity levels had greater values in all of the domains of HRQL related to physical health (i.e., physical function, role limitations due to physical health, bodily pain, and general health) than their more sedentary lifestyle individual's.

In elderly type II diabetic patients, few studies of the health-related quality of life (HRQoL) have been performed. Hiltunen et al. (1996) found that diabetes and impaired glucose tolerance were associated with impaired functional ability in the elderly and that cardio- and cerebrovascular diseases were predictors of this impairment.

In the PAQUID Epidemiological Study (Bourdel-Marchasson et al., 1997), the quality of life was found to be poorer among diabetic subjects, compared with other people of the same age, and they more often had symptoms of ischemic heart disease. The overall PASE scores declined with age regardless of gender, which is consistent with previous research (Washburn et al., 1999).

41

Wexler et al. found that patients with symptomatic co-morbidities such as microvascular complications had a substantially reduced QoL, while those without symptoms showed no reduction of their QoL.

Halaweh H, have shown that active physical activity had a positive effect on both the physical and mental domains of HRQoL among patients with diabetes and the elderly.

Conclusion

In conclusion, healthy older adults who participated in regular physical activity of at least moderate intensity for more than one hour per week had higher values in all eight domains of HRQL than those who were less physically active. It was concluded that the high level of physical activity has a significant effect on all dimensions of the HRQoL in elderly diabetic individuals. The individuals with physically inactive shows the reduced quality of life also. Regular physical activity helps to improve physical and mental functions as well as reverse some effects of chronic disease to keep older people mobile and independent. The evidence shows that regular physical activity is safe for healthy and for frail older people and the risks of developing major cardiovascular and metabolic diseases, obesity, falls, cognitive impairments, osteoporosis and muscular weakness are decreased by regularly completing activities ranging from low intensity walking through to more vigorous sports and resistance exercises.

In this study the result showed the domains of health related quality of life like energy/fatigue and health change shows positive result. The HRQoL of elderly diabetic patients was low who were living in rural areas and with the less physical activity affects the quality of life of elderly diabetic patient. Therefore, incorporating more than one hour of moderate-intensity physical activity each week into the lifestyles of older individuals who are either sedentary or slightly active may improve their HRQL.

References:

1. Bonomi AE, Patrick DL. Validation of the United States version of the World Health Organization Quality of life (WHOQOL) instrument. Journal of Clinical Epidemiology 2000;53(1):19-23.

2. Ragonesi PD, Ragonesi G, Merati L, Taddei MT. The impact of diabetes mellitus on quality of life in elderly patients. Archives of Gerontology and Geriatrics 1998;26(1):417-22.

3. Bagheri H, Ebrahimi H, Taghavi NS, Hassani MR. Evaluation of quality of life in patients with diabetes mellitus based on its complications referred to Emam Hossein Hospital, Shahroud. Journal of Shahrekord University of Medical Sciences 2005;7(2):50-6.

4. Narayan KMV, Boyle JP, Thompson TJ, Sorensen SW, Williamson DF. Lifetime risk for diabetes mellitus in the United States. Journal of American Medical Association 2003;290:1884–90.

5. Mathew A. Mwanyangala, Charles Mayombana, Honorathy Urassa, Jensen Charles, Chrizostom Mahutanga, Salim Abdullah and Rose Nathan, Health status and quality of life among older adults in rural Tanzania. Published: 27 September 2010.

6. Kamlesh joshi, ajit avasthi and rajesh kumar. Health-related quality of life (hrqol) Among the elderly in northern india. Health and Population -Perspectives and Issues 26 (4): 141-153, 2003.

7. Roopa, K.S., and Rama Devi, G. Quality of life of Elderly Diabetic and Hypertensive People – Impact of Intervention Programme. IOSR Journal Of Humanities And Social Science (IOSR-JHSS) Volume 19, Issue 3, Ver. IV (Mar. 2014), PP 67-73.

8. Stumvoll M, Goldstein BJ, van Haeften TW: Type 2 diabetes: principles of pathogenesis and therapy. Lancet, 2005, 365:

1333–1346.

9. Zimmet P, Williams J, de Courten M: Diagnosis and classification of diabetes mellitus. In: Oxford Textbook of Endocrinology and Diabetes. New York: Oxford University Press, 1998, pp 1635–1646.

10. Brassill MJ, O'Sullivan B, O'Halloran D. Levels of physical activity and barriers to exercise in diabetes mellitus. Ir J Med Sci 2010;179 (Suppl 13):S514, http://dx.doi.org/10.1007/s11845-010-0623-y.

11. Luke S Acree, Jessica Longfors. Physical activity is related to quality of life in older adults. Health and Quality of Life Outcomes 2006, 4:37. http://www.hqlo.com/content/4/1/37

12. Stewart KJ, Kelemen MH, Ewart CK: Relationships between selfefficacy and mood before and after exercise training. J Cardiopulm Rehabil 1994, 14:35-42.

13. Stewart AL, King AC, Haskell WL: Endurance exercise and health-related quality of life outcomes in 50–65 year old adults. Gerontologist 1993, 33:782-789.

14. Washburn, R. A., McAuley, E., Katula, J., Mihalko, S. L., & Boileau, R. A. (1999). The physical activity scale for the elderly (PASE): Evidence for validity. Journal of Clinical Epidemiology, 52(7), 643-651.

15. 23. Wexler DJ, Grant RW, Wittenberg E, Bosch JL, Cagliero E, Delahanty L, Blais MA, Meigs JB. Correlates of health-related quality of life in type 2 diabetes. Diabetologia. 2006;49:1489–97.

16. Halaweh H, Willen C, Grimby-Ekman A, et al. Physical Activity and Health-Related Quality of Life Among Community Dwelling Elderly. J Clin Med Res 2015;7:845–52.

17. Cho KO. The Positive Effect of Physical Activity on Health and Health-related Quality of Life in Elderly Korean People-Evidence from the Fifth Korea National Health and Nutrition Examination Survey. J Lifestyle Med 2014;4:86–94.

Pamphlet for the exercise

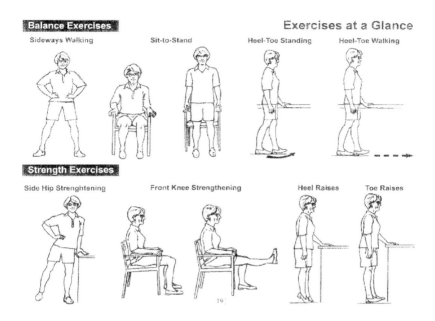

Balance Exercises   Exercises at a Glance

Sideways Walking   Sit-to-Stand   Heel-Toe Standing   Heel-Toe Walking

Strength Exercises

Side Hip Strenghtening   Front Knee Strengthening   Heel Raises   Toe Raises

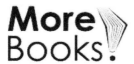
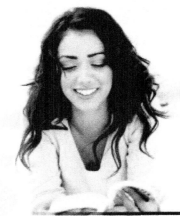
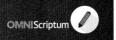

Printed in Great Britain
by Amazon

83423219R00037